AF800789

NCCN Guidelines for Patients®

The essential guide for people facing cancer.

Based on care recommendations from leading cancer experts.

Explains high-quality cancer care provided at state-of-the-art cancer centers.

Reviewed and revised every year.

Did you know that top cancer centers across the United States work together to improve cancer care? This alliance of leading cancer centers is called the National Comprehensive Cancer Network® (NCCN®).

Because cancer care is always evolving, NCCN develops and frequently updates evidence-based cancer care recommendations used by health care providers worldwide. These recommendations are known as the NCCN Clinical Practice Guidelines in Oncology (NCCN Guidelines®).

The NCCN Guidelines for Patients plainly explain these expert recommendations, so you can talk with your care team about the best care for you.

These NCCN Guidelines for Patients are based on the NCCN Guidelines® for Prostate Cancer Early Detection, Version 2.2026 — February 18, 2026.

View the NCCN Guidelines for Patients free online: NCCN.org/patientguidelines

Find an NCCN Cancer Center near you: NCCN.org/cancercenters

Learn how the NCCN Guidelines for Patients are developed: NCCN.org/patient-guidelines-process

Connect with us

@NCCNorg @NCCNVideo NCCN @NCCNorg

Supporters

NATIONAL COMPREHENSIVE CANCER NETWORK®
NCCN FOUNDATION
Guiding Treatment. Changing Lives.

NCCN Guidelines for Patients are supported by funding from the NCCN Foundation®

NCCN Foundation gratefully acknowledges the following supporters for helping to make available these NCCN Guidelines for Patients: AstraZeneca and Novartis Pharmaceuticals Corporation.

NCCN independently adapts, updates, and hosts the NCCN Guidelines for Patients. Our corporate supporters do not participate in the development of the NCCN Guidelines for Patients and are not responsible for the content and recommendations contained therein.

To make a gift, visit
NCCNFoundation.org/Donate

To learn more, visit online
NCCN.org/patientguidelines
or email
PatientGuidelines@NCCN.org

Contents

NCCN Foundation seeks to support the millions of patients and their families affected by a cancer diagnosis by funding and distributing NCCN Guidelines for Patients. NCCN Foundation is also committed to advancing cancer treatment by funding the nation's promising doctors at the center of innovation in cancer research. For more details and the full library of patient and caregiver resources, visit NCCN.org/patients.

National Comprehensive Cancer Network (NCCN) and NCCN Foundation
3025 Chemical Road, Suite 100, Plymouth Meeting, PA 19462 USA

1

About prostate cancer screening

Anyone with a prostate is at risk for prostate cancer. Screening tests can help find prostate cancer early, when it's more treatable. This guide will help you talk with your doctor and care team about whether prostate cancer screening is right for you.

What is prostate cancer screening?

Prostate cancer screening is testing to find cancer early, before it can get worse and cause symptoms.

Prostate cancer found at an earlier stage is usually treated more easily and more successfully than prostate cancer found at an advanced stage.

That's why screening is so important. Detecting prostate cancer early helps to prevent advanced cancer, which may cause pain, serious illness, or death.

However, many cases of prostate cancer never become advanced. That's because most prostate cancers grow slowly, don't cause symptoms, and usually don't need treatment.

Prostate cancer screening aims to avoid detecting these slow-growing cancers because finding them may lead to unnecessary treatment, harmful complications, and needless worry.

Keep in mind that most people who are screened have a normal result with no sign of prostate cancer—which can bring peace of mind.

The prostate gland is an important part of the male reproductive system. It's located in the pelvis just below the bladder.

The prostate is the size of a ping-pong ball in a young adult. It grows larger with age.

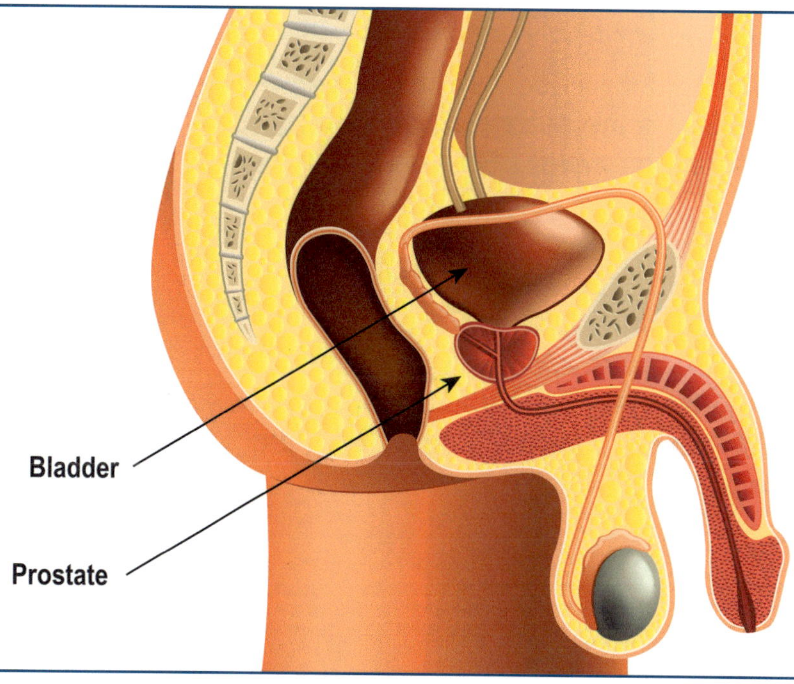

What is the prostate?

The prostate gland is an important part of the male sexual reproductive system. This system also includes the penis, seminal vesicles, and testicles.

The prostate is located just below the bladder in the pelvis, deep inside the area of your body between your hip bones. It's about the size of a ping-pong ball when you're a young adult. It naturally grows larger with age.

The prostate is 1 of the body's important glands. A gland is an organ that makes fluids or chemicals the body needs.

The prostate gland makes a protein (prostate-specific antigen, or PSA) that helps semen transport sperm.

The prostate also contains muscles that help propel semen through the male organs during ejaculation.

What is prostate cancer?

Prostate cancer is the second most common cancer in American males. (Skin cancer is the first.)

Prostate cancer occurs when something goes wrong with the natural processes of cells in the prostate. The cells develop genetic changes (mutations) that allow them to multiply and grow out of control. These abnormal cells are cancer cells.

Cancer cells can crowd out and replace normal cells. They can also spread outside of the prostate to nearby areas or further parts of the body. This can end up causing significant symptoms and can even be life-threatening.

Prostate cancer can be very different from person to person. For many, prostate cancer grows slowly—so slowly that it doesn't spread, cause symptoms, or need to be treated.

But for some, prostate cancer grows quickly and causes difficult symptoms. Fast-growing prostate cancer or prostate cancer that's likely to spread often needs to be treated.

Do I need to be screened for prostate cancer?

Even though prostate cancer can occur in anyone with a prostate, not everyone with a prostate needs or wants to be screened for prostate cancer.

Screening is generally recommended to begin at **age 45** if you have an **average risk** for prostate cancer.

Screening is recommended at **age 40** if you have a **higher risk** for prostate cancer. Factors linked to higher risk include your health, race, and whether you have family members who've had prostate cancer or other cancers. These factors are explained in *Chapter 2: Who needs to be screened for prostate cancer?*

But there's another factor to consider. Screening for prostate cancer isn't always harmless. Screening has risks as well as benefits.

Learning more about prostate cancer screening can help. NCCN experts recommend that anyone wondering about prostate cancer screening should:

- Understand what's involved in screening
- Weigh the risk and benefits of screening
- Talk with their doctor to discuss whether screening is right for them

This guide can help you decide whether prostate cancer screening is right for you.

The goal of prostate cancer screening is to detect aggressive cancer that could be life-threatening. But screening may find harmless slow-growing cancer that only needs to be watched.

What's involved in prostate cancer screening?

Screening for prostate cancer involves a blood test and, sometimes, a brief physical exam.

PSA test

The main screening test for prostate cancer is a blood test that measures the amount of PSA in your bloodstream.

A PSA level that's above average for your age group means that you have a higher risk for prostate cancer. The higher your PSA level, the greater the risk.

A higher PSA also increases the risk for prostate cancer that's more aggressive—in other words, prostate cancer that's often harder to treat.

But many things besides prostate cancer can raise your PSA level. So if screening finds that your PSA is higher than normal, you should have a few more tests that can confirm or rule out prostate cancer. You can learn about further tests in *Chapter 3: What to expect at a prostate cancer screening?*

Prostate exam

Another part of prostate cancer screening that some doctors recommend is a prostate exam. Also called a digital rectal exam, the prostate exam checks the size and texture of your prostate gland for signs of cancer.

For this test, your doctor will insert a gloved finger into your rear end (rectum) to feel your prostate gland for anything unusual. An irregular or hardened part of the prostate could be a sign of cancer.

A prostate exam is not always necessary, and you can refuse it if you don't want it.

The PSA test and prostate exam are explained more fully in *Chapter 3: What to expect at a prostate cancer screening?*

How can I get the best care?

Advocate for yourself. You have an important role to play in your care. Many people feel more satisfied when they actively take part in planning their cancer screening.

The NCCN Guidelines for Patients will help you play a larger role in your care. Discuss the recommendations in this guide with your care team. Ask questions about your options and share your goals and concerns.

Don't know what to ask? You're not alone. That's why we include suggested questions to ask at the end of chapters.

Keep reading to find the best option for you.

How this guide can help you

Making decisions about cancer care is stressful. There's a lot to learn, and you don't know what the future holds.

Use this guide to get the information and support you need.

Patients, doctors, and other health care professionals trust the NCCN Guidelines for Patients. This guide uses clear, everyday language to explain current cancer screening recommendations made by respected experts in the field. Their recommendations are based on the latest research and practices at leading cancer centers.

Your health is unique to you, so your cancer care should be, too. As you read this guide, you'll learn which options are likely to provide the best results for you. And you'll be better prepared to talk with your care team

2

Who needs to be screened for prostate cancer?

There's a lot of information out there about prostate cancer. It can be difficult to make sense of it all. This chapter specifies who should be screened for prostate cancer. Other chapters provide reliable guidance about when and how often to be screened.

Anyone with a prostate—depending on their health, age, and risk factors—should consider having prostate cancer screening.

The goal of prostate cancer screening is to identify cancer long before it would cause symptoms. As such, a person's health and life expectancy are very important to consider when deciding whether to have screening.

Older age, in fact, is the leading risk factor for prostate cancer. A risk factor is anything that increases your chance for getting a disease.

Other risk factors for prostate cancer include Black race, a family history of cancer, inherited genetic changes, and being exposed to Agent Orange.

Risk factors don't necessarily cause cancer. But people with prostate cancer may have 1 or more of these risk factors.

Older age

Age is the most important risk factor for prostate cancer. The older you are, the greater your chance for developing it.

Prostate cancer is diagnosed most often in people aged 65 years of age and over. But that doesn't mean you should wait until you're 65 or over to be screened.

Older age is the most important risk factor for prostate cancer. A risk factor is something that increases your chance for getting a disease.

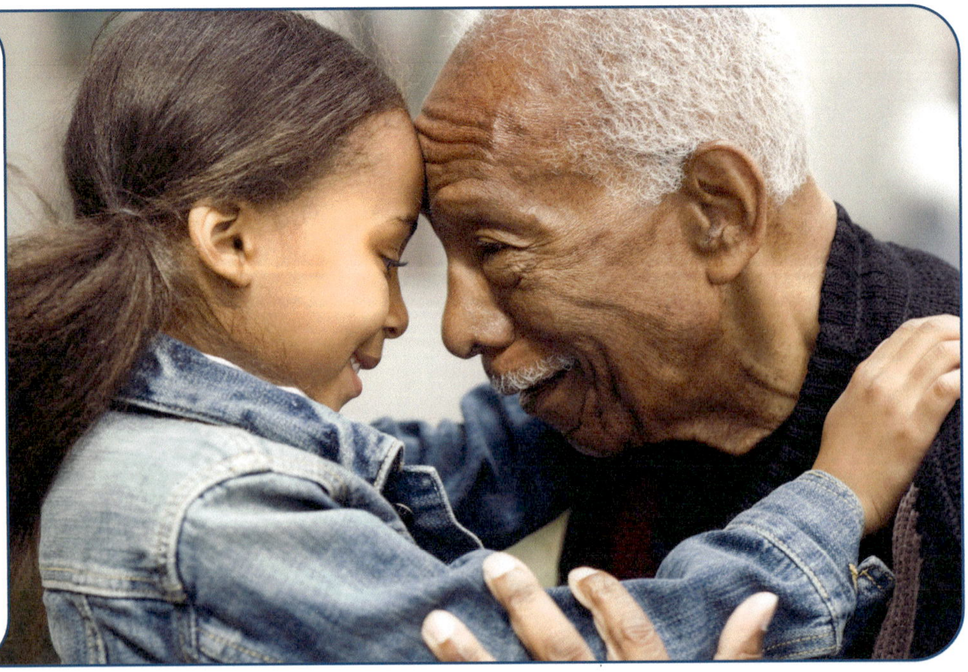

The recommended age to have your first screening depends on whether you have any risk factors. See **Guide 1**.

No risk factors

NCCN experts recommend that individuals with no risk factors have their first screening for prostate cancer by **age 45.**

One or more risk factors

People with any risk factors have a greater chance for developing prostate cancer. NCCN experts recommend they talk to their doctor about getting screened beginning at **age 40.** (Prostate cancer is uncommon under age 40.)

Is there an age when you no longer need prostate cancer screening?

Most individuals can safely discontinue prostate cancer screening at **age 75.** That's because people at this age have a very low chance for developing prostate cancer that becomes advanced in their lifetime.

It's true that some individuals age 75 and over will develop low-grade prostate cancer. But it isn't likely to shorten their lives or compromise their health. Finding these cancers can lead to unnecessary treatment that doesn't help and may be harmful. So experts don't recommend screening in this age group.

Guide 1
When to start prostate cancer screening based on your age and risk factors

	Risk factors					
Age	**None**	**Black/ African American ancestry**	**Family history of prostate cancer**	**Your history of cancer**	**Inherited genetic changes**	**Agent Orange exposure**
Under 40						
40 to 45		✓	✓	✓	✓	✓
45 to 75	✓	✓	✓	✓	✓	✓
Over 75*						

These are general recommendations. Consider your individual circumstances.
*Prostate cancer screening over age 75 is recommended only for very healthy individuals who expect to live another 10 or more years.

There are some exceptions. If you're 75 years of age or over, you might still consider screening if you:

- Have a high or rising PSA level
- Have a possible tumor as detected by a prostate exam or MRI scan
- Are very healthy and are expected to live another 10 or more years

Of course, you can always talk with your doctor about prostate cancer screening no matter your age.

Black race

Black males in the United States are more likely to develop prostate cancer than other males. Prostate cancer in Black males is also more likely to occur at an earlier age and be more aggressive and more advanced when diagnosed.

What's more, Black males are almost twice as likely to die of prostate cancer than other males.

Several things contribute to these differences, such as biological factors, barriers to accessing health care (including screening), and other social and clinical considerations. Researchers are trying to figure out the reasons for these differences and what can be done to improve outcomes.

In light of these concerns, many experts recommend Black males talk to their doctors about getting screening tests earlier and more often than what's recommended for those at average risk.

Specifically, Black males are encouraged to have prostate cancer screening at 40 years of age and to continue to be screened regularly from then on.

Anyone with a risk for prostate cancer should consider prostate cancer screening.

Risks for prostate cancer are higher in people with older age, Black race, a family history of cancer, inherited genetic changes, or exposure to Agent Orange.

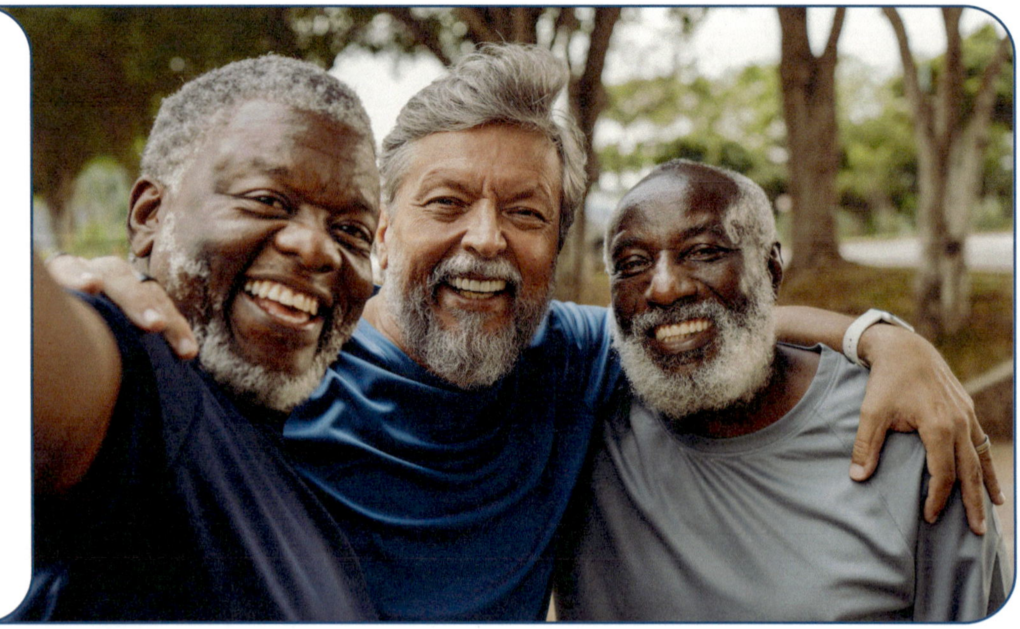

Cancer in your family

The information about the diseases and health conditions in your family is called your family medical history, or simply family history.

A family history may reflect a pattern of certain diseases among family members. Having a close family member with prostate cancer (a sibling or parent) increases the chance for getting it yourself.

People with a family history of certain cancers (prostate, breast, ovarian, pancreatic, and others) may also be at higher risk for prostate cancer. Patients with a family history of these cancers should consider asking their doctors about genetic testing.

Inherited genetic changes

An inherited genetic change isn't a common cause of prostate cancer. As explained in Chapter 1, most cases of prostate cancer occur from cells that develop genetic changes (mutations) all on their own.

But sometimes, genetic changes can be passed down from a parent to a child. For instance, having an inherited genetic change in the *BRCA1* or *BRCA2* gene may increase your risk for getting prostate cancer as well as other cancers.

These genetic changes—also called variants—can also raise the risk for prostate cancer that develops at an earlier age (under age 50) and is more aggressive.

“No one ever said to me prostate cancer is something that hits African American men harder and earlier. That's why I was shocked when they told me I had it. We [African Americans] are warned about heart disease and diabetes, not prostate cancer.”

More information on inherited genetic changes can be found in *NCCN Guidelines for Patients: Genetic Testing for Hereditary Breast, Ovarian, Pancreatic, and Prostate Cancers*, available at NCCN.org/patientguidelines and on the NCCN Patient Guides for Cancer.

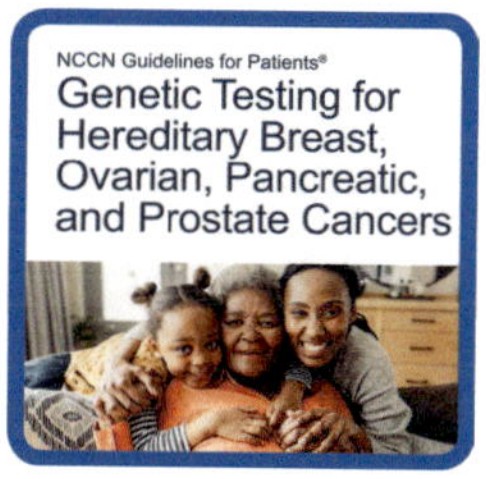

Chemical exposure

Being exposed to Agent Orange may be associated with an increased risk for advanced prostate cancer as well as other cancers.

Agent Orange was a chemical sprayed by the U.S. military during the Vietnam war to get rid of plants, trees, and crops. Since then, Agent Orange and other herbicides have been linked to numerous illnesses and cancers, including prostate cancer, among Vietnam war veterans and Vietnamese people.

Key points

- A risk factor is anything that increases your chance for getting a disease. But risk factors don't necessarily cause cancer.
- Risk factors for prostate cancer include age, Black race, a family history of cancer, inherited genetic changes, and being exposed to Agent Orange.
- People who have 1 or more risk factors for prostate cancer have a greater chance for developing it. These individuals should consider getting screened starting at age 40.
- Individuals who have no risk factors should get a prostate cancer screening starting at 45 years of age.
- Age 75 is a safe cutoff for prostate cancer screening for most individuals.

Questions to ask

- What are my risks for getting prostate cancer?
- At what age should I start prostate cancer screening?
- At what age should I stop prostate cancer screening?
- Are my chances for getting prostate cancer greater if I have more risk factors?

"Be your own advocate. Talk to someone who has gone through the same thing as you. Ask a lot of questions, even the ones you are afraid to ask."

What's next?

This chapter explained the risk factors for prostate cancer. The next chapter describes the screening process itself so you'll know what to expect.

3

What to expect at a prostate cancer screening?

You may be surprised to learn how quick and easy a prostate cancer screening really is. It mainly involves a simple blood test. Depending on the results of your blood test, you may need further testing and evaluation.

Chapter 1 introduced the tests that make up a prostate cancer screening. You also learned about the risk factors for prostate cancer in Chapter 2. Now, it's time you find out exactly what happens at a screening.

A prostate cancer screening is mainly an ordinary blood test for a substance called PSA. Sometimes it includes a prostate exam, too.

PSA test

Prostate-specific antigen (PSA) is a protein made inside of the prostate gland. Its job is to help semen transport sperm. All prostate cells, both normal cells and cancer cells, make PSA.

While most PSA goes into semen, a little bit ends up in the bloodstream, too. A PSA test measures the amount of PSA in your bloodstream.

As with an ordinary blood test, a nurse, physician assistant, or phlebotomist will insert a needle into your arm to collect a small sample of your blood.

This can be done in less than 15 minutes at your primary care doctor's office, a urologist's office, or a local walk-in testing lab. It can also be done with other routine blood work your doctor obtains. You don't need to fast the night before.

A PSA test is a simple blood test. A high level of PSA in your blood may be a sign of prostate cancer.

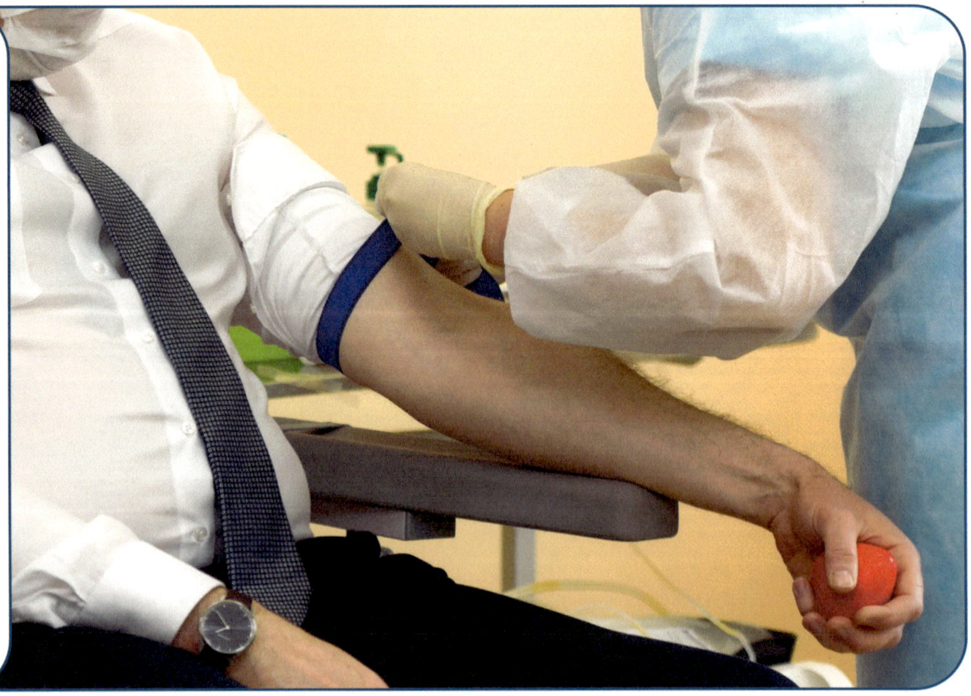

Your blood sample will be tested to measure the amount of PSA in your blood. PSA level (also called total PSA) is measured in nanograms of PSA per milliliter (ng/mL) of blood.

If there's something wrong with the prostate, it can release more PSA into the bloodstream.

An unusually high amount of PSA in the blood may be a sign of prostate cancer. The higher the amount of PSA in your blood, the greater is your risk for prostate cancer.

However, a high PSA doesn't cause prostate cancer. In fact, most individuals with higher PSA levels don't have prostate cancer. That's because age and other factors—such as an enlarged prostate or a urinary tract infection—also cause high levels of PSA.

Indeed, your PSA level also increases with age.

This means that a PSA test by itself can't provide a diagnosis of prostate cancer. So the PSA test is often paired with imaging or a prostate exam, or both, to decide whether you need further testing.

> **"We take better care of our cars and our lawns than we take care of ourselves. So think of it like this: Screening for prostate cancer is preventive maintenance."**

Some prescription and over-the-counter medicines and supplements can also change your PSA level, causing a false result. See **Guide 2**.

Before your PSA test, let your doctor or health care team know about any medicines or supplements you're taking.

Guide 2
Medicines that may affect PSA

Prescription medicine	**Raises ↑ or lowers ↓ PSA**
Dutasteride (Avodart)	↓ PSA
Finasteride (Propecia, Proscar)	↓ PSA

Prostate exam

A prostate exam is a way to check the size and texture of your prostate gland. An irregular or hardened part of the prostate could be a sign of a tumor.

A prostate exam is also called a digital rectal exam. The word digital refers to a finger (digit). Your doctor will insert a gloved and lubricated finger into your rectum to feel your prostate for any signs of cancer. This is possible because the rectum is right next to the prostate.

Not all parts of the prostate can be felt during a prostate exam, though. So it's paired with a PSA test and other factors—your age, race, family history, and more—to determine whether you need further testing.

For many years, people have avoided prostate screening because they didn't want a prostate exam. Although the exam isn't painful, it can be embarrassing, awkward, and unpleasant. But it usually takes only a few seconds. Try to relax and breathe, which can make it less uncomfortable.

NCCN experts say a prostate exam, if one is performed, is most useful for individuals who have a higher PSA level.

Nowadays, a prostate exam is no longer required. Also, some doctors don't recommend a prostate exam because it's not very good at finding cancer on its own, so they may recommend an MRI of the prostate instead.

Then again, on rare occasions, a prostate exam detects a potential tumor that a PSA test doesn't.

The choice to have it is up to you, based on shared decision-making with your doctor.

Prostate exam

A prostate exam is a procedure in which your doctor inserts a finger into your rectum to feel your prostate. An irregular or hardened part of the prostate could be a sign of a tumor.

Not all parts of the prostate can be felt during this exam, though. So other tests, like PSA level and imaging, are used to get a more complete picture of your prostate health.

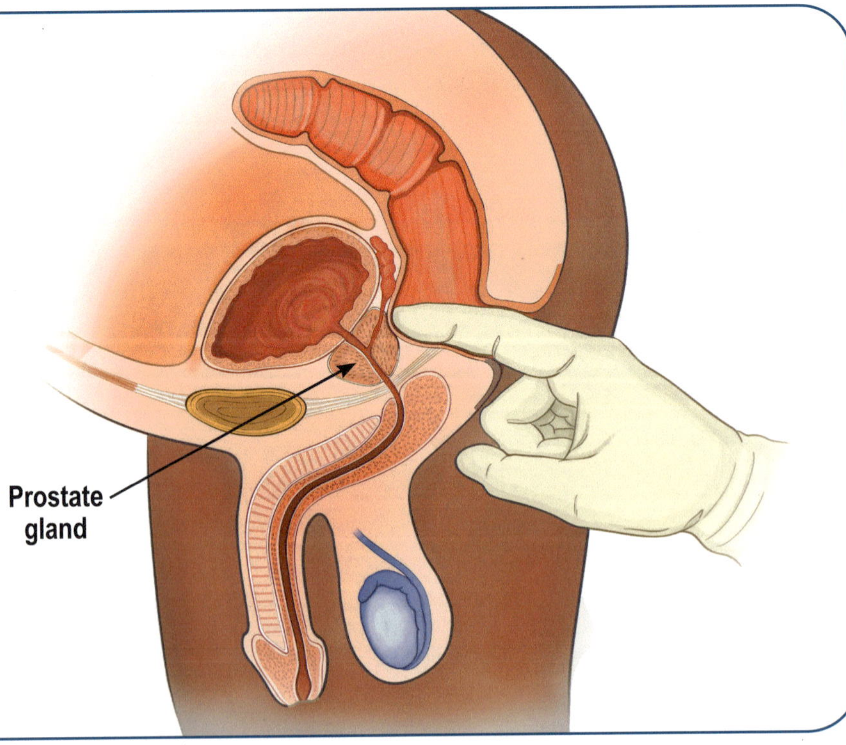

What happens after a screening?

After your prostate screening, your blood sample will be sent to a lab for testing. The test results are usually available within a few days.

What happens next depends on your test result. Also see **Guide 3**.

Test result: PSA is normal

If your PSA level is normal for your age and your prostate exam is also normal (if you had one), then all is well. You don't need to do anything further for now.

Your doctor will likely recommend you have prostate cancer screenings about every 2 years, or more or less often:

- **More often** (every 1 to 2 years) if you have any risk factors
- **Less often** (every 2 to 4 years) if your PSA level is very low and you have no risk factors

Test result: PSA is higher than normal

If your PSA level is higher than normal for your age, you'll likely need further testing and evaluation to find out if there is any cancer in your prostate.

A high PSA level doesn't mean you definitely have prostate cancer. Rather, it's a red flag that signals the need for further testing and evaluation. Turn to the next chapter to learn about further testing and evaluation.

How to prepare for a prostate cancer screening

- **Be prepared to describe your family history.**
  It's helpful to know if any close relatives on both sides of your family had cancer or other health issues. If so, know the specific type of cancer, where the cancer started, if it was in multiple locations, and if your relative had genetic testing.
- **Tell your doctor or health care team if you take any prescription or over-the-counter medicines, herbals, or supplements.**
  Some medicines and supplements can affect your PSA level, which can cause incorrect test results.
- **Find out if there's a cost for screening.**
  Medicare and most health insurance plans pay for at least 1 prostate cancer screening per year.

Guide 3
What happens after a prostate cancer screening?

Your risk factors	Your screening result		Your next steps
No risk factors	Very low PSA (less than 1 ng/mL)	→	Continue prostate screening every 2 to 4 years
	Slightly elevated PSA (1 to 3 ng/mL)	→	Continue prostate screening every 1 to 2 years
	Elevated PSA (more than 3 ng/mL) **and/or** your prostate exam suggests a strong possibility of cancer	→	Have a second PSA test to verify the initial PSA. You'll need further testing with MRI and possibly a biopsy.
One or more risk factors	Low to slightly elevated PSA (3 ng/mL or under)	→	Continue prostate screening every 1 or 2 years. If you are in your 40s and have an elevated PSA, you may need further testing with MRI and possibly a biopsy.
	Elevated PSA (more than 3 ng/mL) **and/or** your prostate exam suggests a strong possibility of cancer	→	Have a second PSA test to verify the initial PSA. You'll need further testing with MRI and possibly a biopsy.
Whether you have or don't have risk factors	Low PSA **but** your prostate exam suggests a strong possibility of cancer	→	Further testing with MRI and possibly a biopsy.

Key points

- Prostate-specific antigen (PSA) is a protein made inside of the prostate gland. All prostate cells, both normal cells and cancer cells, make PSA.
- A PSA test measures the amount of PSA in your bloodstream. An unusually high amount of PSA in the blood may be a sign of prostate cancer.
- A PSA test by itself can't diagnose cancer because age and other factors can also cause PSA to rise.
- If a PSA test finds that your PSA level is higher than normal, you'll likely need further testing and evaluation to find out if you have prostate cancer.
- A prostate exam, also called a digital rectal exam, checks the size and texture of the prostate gland for any sign of a tumor.
- A prostate exam frequently misses cancers because not all parts of the prostate can be felt during the exam.
- A prostate exam is not always necessary. But if one is performed, it's most useful for individuals who have a higher PSA level.

Questions to ask

- Can any of the medicines I'm taking affect my PSA level?
- Is there any way I can reduce my risk for prostate cancer?
- Can I just have the PSA test and skip the prostate exam?
- Will my risk factors affect the results of the screening?

What's next?

Prostate cancer screening can't provide a definitive result, and you and your health will continue to change. For that reason, if your PSA is normal for your age, you should continue to have prostate cancer screenings on a regular basis after your've had an initial screening. If your PSA is elevated, see the next chapter to learn what further testing is available beyond a screening.

4

Further testing and evaluation

If your prostate cancer screening showed your PSA is higher than normal, it could be due to something other than cancer. Before undergoing a biopsy, you should have further testing and evaluation to get more information to make sure you need a biopsy.

What is shared decision-making?

Your doctor and health care team can help you decide whether a biopsy—or a prostate cancer screening, for that matter—is right for you.

This doesn't mean they'll take the responsibility for the decision off your hands. Rather, you'll work together to figure out the best decision for you.

This is called shared decision-making.

Your doctor is the expert on cancer diagnosis and treatment. You are the expert on **you**—your body, values, priorities, and goals.

Shared decision-making is when you work together with your doctors and care team to create a plan that fits both your medical needs and your personal goals.

Shared decision-making involves 4 key tasks. Together, you, your doctor, and your care team will:

1. Share information with each other.
2. Each have a say in the decision-making process.
3. Consider both the medical concerns and your personal values and goals.
4. Make a joint decision on what to do.

Shared decision-making is when you work together with your doctors and care team to create a plan that fits both your medical needs and your personal goals.

Make the most of shared decision-making to reach a decision that's right for you.

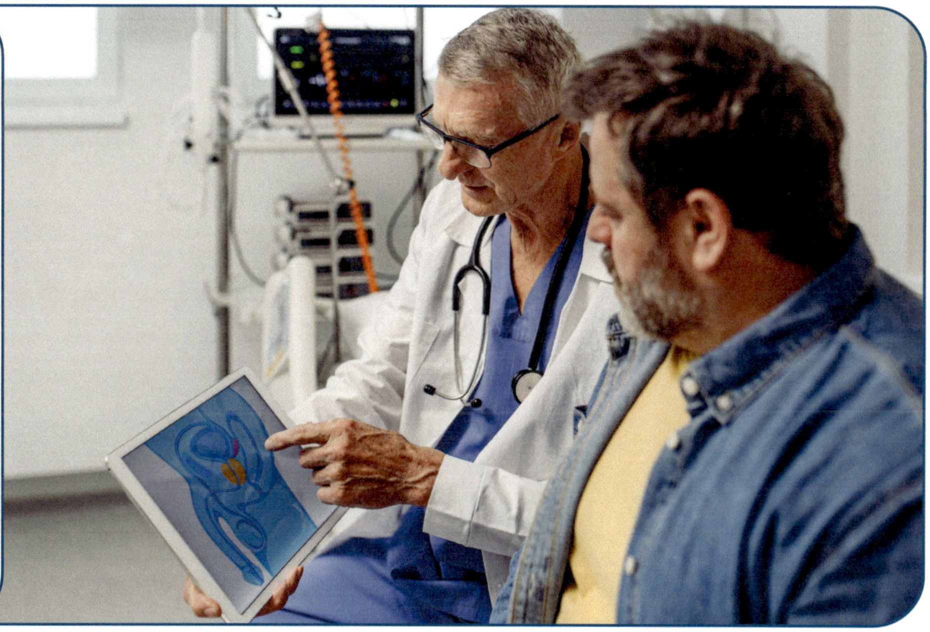

Further testing before biopsy

In the past, having an elevated level of prostate-specific antigen (PSA) often led directly to a biopsy. Although a biopsy is still the only way to diagnose cancer, it's also an invasive procedure with risks of its own.

Nowadays, experts often recommend having additional noninvasive tests, particularly an MRI scan, before going ahead with a biopsy.

Further testing after a prostate screening includes another PSA test, a prostate exam, and an evaluation for benign (non-cancer) causes.

Another PSA test

You'll have a second PSA test a few weeks after your initial screening. This is done to make sure the result of the first PSA test wasn't an error.

After your second PSA test:

- If your PSA is still at a higher level, you may need to have an MRI and/or a biopsy.
- If your PSA has increased a lot from your initial screening or it has increased in a short amount of time, these may be signs of aggressive cancer. You should have an MRI and a biopsy.
- If your PSA level has gone down to a normal level, your doctor will recommend when to have your next prostate cancer screening.

Prostate exam

If you didn't have a prostate exam at your initial screening, you may have one now.

If your initial PSA test finds that your level is higher than normal, you should have a second PSA test a few weeks later to confirm the result of the first test.

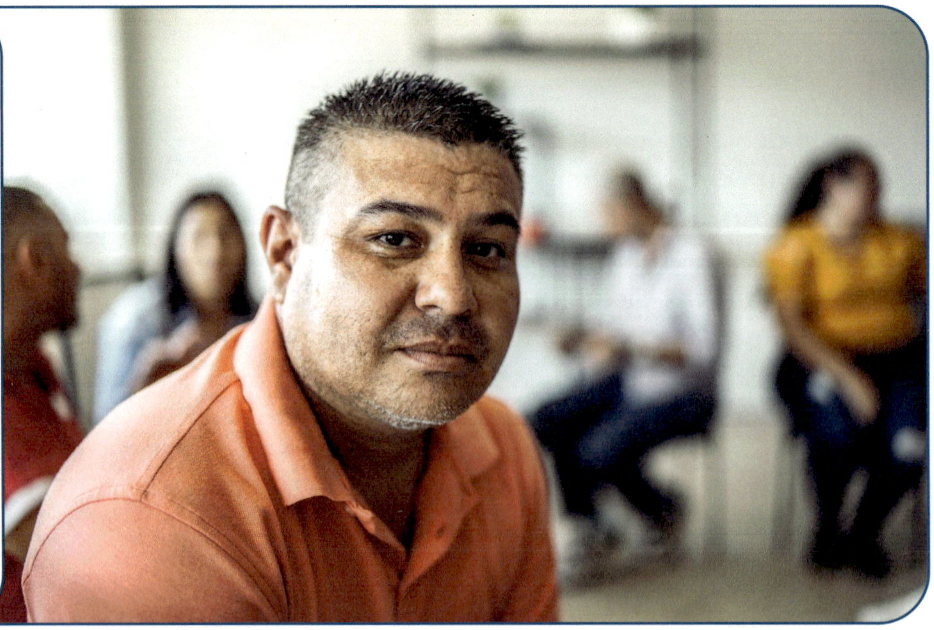

Checking for non-cancer causes

Many reasons besides cancer can cause your PSA to rise. Before going any further, your doctor will check you for:

- **Infection** – Urinary tract infections and other types of infection can cause inflammation of the prostate (prostatitis), which can raise your PSA level.
- **Enlarged prostate** – Enlargement of the prostate, also called benign prostatic hyperplasia, occurs naturally with age. The larger the prostate, the more PSA it can release.

If your PSA is elevated due to something other than cancer, your doctor will diagnose and address the problem. But be aware that you may still be at risk for prostate cancer. In other words, you can have both an enlarged prostate and prostate cancer at the same time.

Also be aware that an enlarged prostate doesn't cause prostate cancer.

If other causes of cancer aren't apparent, your doctor will likely recommend you have an MRI and/or a biopsy to find out what's going on.

MRI before biopsy

If your PSA is elevated, your doctor may recommend you have an MRI scan before you undergo a biopsy.

An MRI can show the size of your prostate as well as areas of possible prostate cancer. It can also help you avoid getting a biopsy unnecessarily.

Have an MRI first

MRI is a type of imaging that takes pictures (images) of the inside of the body. An MRI scanner is a large machine with a tunnel in

An MRI scan can detect aggressive, fast-growing cancer in the prostate. This is the kind that should be biopsied.

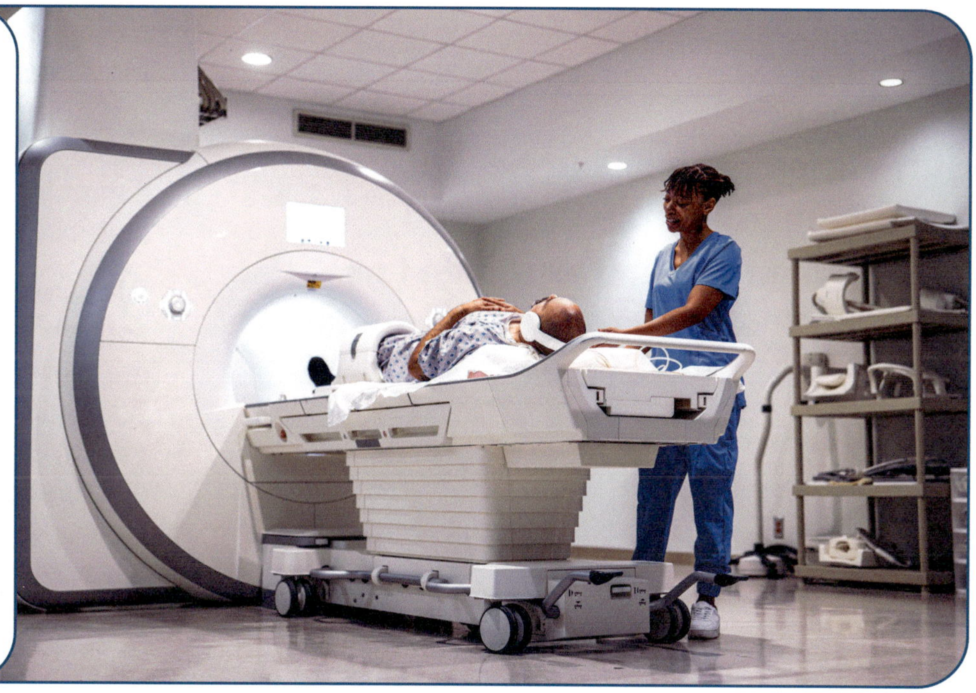

the middle. It uses radio waves and powerful magnets to provide a detailed view within the prostate.

An MRI scan of the prostate can help decide whether or not a biopsy is needed. That's because it can help detect aggressive, fast-growing prostate cancer—the kind that should be biopsied.

If the MRI shows nothing suspicious, it usually means a biopsy won't be necessary.

An advanced type of MRI that's used for prostate cancer is called multiparametric MRI, or mpMRI. This kind of MRI combines several imaging techniques that improve its ability to identify aggressive prostate cancer.

If you're expected to have a biopsy, mpMRI can improve the accuracy by pinpointing suspicious areas of the prostate for the biopsy to target.

"Stay curious about your health, learn from trusted sources, find your community, and advocate for yourself. These simple actions might just save your life—I believe they saved mine."

It's important to know that mpMRI, like most medical tests, isn't perfect. It occasionally misses an area of cancer (a false-negative result).

Or it may detect something that looks like cancer but actually isn't (a false-positive).

Also, mpMRI is not available at every hospital or clinic. You might have another type of MRI, such as biparametric MRI (bpMRI), instead.

Have other non-invasive tests, if needed

In addition to an MRI, other tests can help determine whether a biopsy is necessary. Not everyone will receive all of these tests.

- **PSA density** – This measurement can identify when someone's high PSA level is caused by an enlarged prostate rather than prostate cancer. It can help these individuals avoid unnecessary biopsies.
- **Risk calculators** – A risk calculator is an online tool that incorporates your clinical information—your age, race, family cancer history, PSA level, and so on—to estimate your risk for cancer that can be detected by a biopsy. It can also estimate your risk for having aggressive, high-risk cancer.
- **Biomarker tests** – A biomarker is something in your body that can be measured to provide information about your health. Biomarker tests for prostate cancer analyze samples of your blood or urine to look for molecular or genetic biomarkers linked to prostate cancer.

Review all of your results

Together, you, your doctor, and your care team will review the results of your prostate screening and any other tests you've had up to this point, particularly an MRI.

Altogether, this clinical information will give you a good idea whether your prostate is likely or isn't likely to have detectable cancer.

Doctors often refer to this likelihood as suspicion of cancer. In this sense, a suspicion isn't just a hunch or intuition—it's based on hard evidence, such as your test results, risk factors, and any other clinical information that's been gathered.

A low suspicion of prostate cancer means that significant cancer **isn't likely.** A high suspicion means prostate cancer **is likely**.

If prostate cancer isn't likely

If significant prostate cancer doesn't seem likely (low suspicion), you can say no to a biopsy, based on shared decision-making with your doctor and care team.

Of course, this doesn't mean you can ignore your prostate altogether. It's recommended you have another screening in 6 to 12 months. And you should continue to have regular prostate screenings from then on.

Keep in mind that you may indeed have low-grade, slow-growing prostate cancer despite low suspicion. But also keep in mind that it's causing no symptoms and is not likely to affect your health or reduce your lifespan.

It's unlikely that low-grade prostate cancer will become more serious. But if it does, it can be caught at one of your regular prostate screenings before it can cause harm.

Many people who are interested in learning more about prostate cancer screening find it helpful to talk with others who have the same questions or have gone through screening.

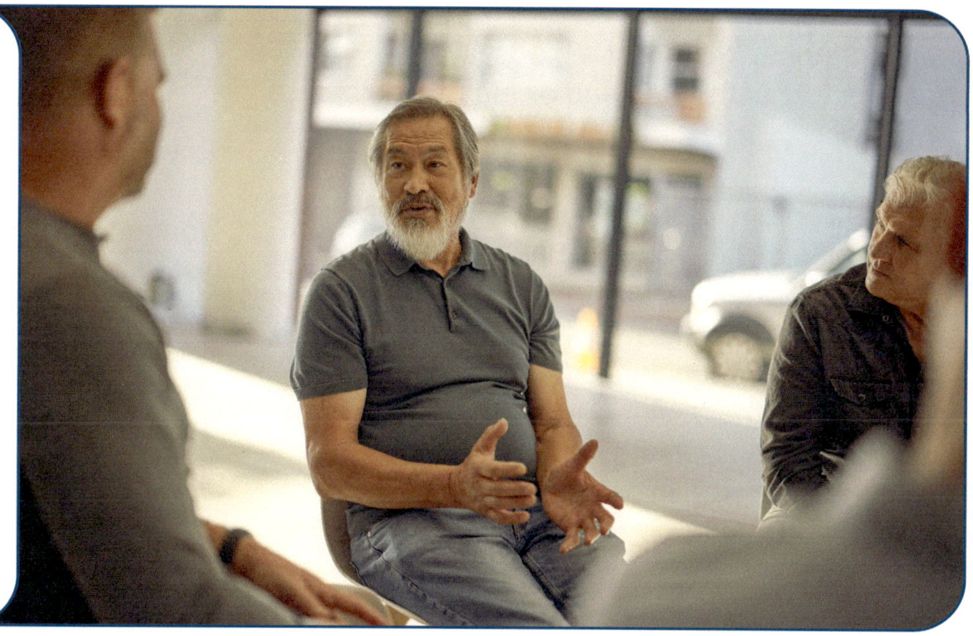

If prostate cancer is likely

If the results of your PSA test(s) and other assessments indicate that a biopsy is likely to detect prostate cancer (high suspicion), it's generally recommended to go ahead and have a biopsy.

Biopsy

Although MRI technology is getting better at detecting areas of the prostate that look like cancer, it still can't identify cancer for certain.

The only way to diagnose prostate cancer is with a biopsy.

A biopsy is a procedure in which a sample of cells or tissue is removed from the body and tested for cancer cells.

It's important to know that a biopsy won't cause cancer cells to spread or make prostate cancer worse.

Biopsies can be done in a surgical center or in a doctor's office. You'll be under sedation or receive local anesthesia to numb the pain.

Using imaging for guidance (ultrasound, MRI, or both), the doctor will insert a hollow needle either through the rectum or through the perineum (the skin between the anus and scrotum) and into the prostate gland. When the needle is removed, it will pull out a small sample of prostate tissue. At least 12 or more samples will be removed from various parts of the prostate.

After the biopsy, the tissue samples will be examined by a pathologist and tested for cancer cells.

What happens next depends on your biopsy result. It can take a week or 2 to receive your biopsy results.

Biopsy result: Cancer is found

If cancer cells are found in your biopsy samples, you may hear this called a positive result. This means the biopsy **did** find cancer—it was "positive" for cancer.

A diagnosis of cancer can bring a rollercoaster of emotions. Shock, anxiety, frustration, and even denial are all common. Sharing your results with family, friends, or a therapist can help.

Taking an active, problem-solving approach can also be useful. You can try stress management techniques, learn more about your prostate cancer, or do other activities to keep your mind and body busy while you talk to your doctor and care team about next steps.

Your doctor or another clinician will be able to estimate the amount of cancer in the prostate and how aggressive it may be, based on the appearance of the cancer cells under the microscope, your PSA, and your MRI findings. This information is vital for developing a treatment plan.

You can read more about diagnosis and treatment for prostate cancer in *NCCN Guidelines for Patients: Early-Stage Prostate Cancer* and the *NCCN Guidelines for Patients: Advanced-Stage Prostate Cancer*, available at NCCN.org/patientguidelines and on the NCCN Patient Guides for Cancer app.

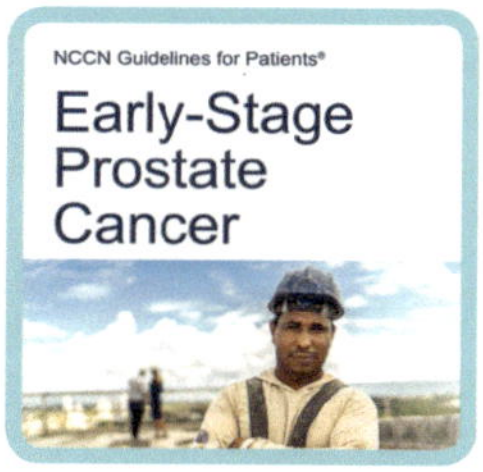

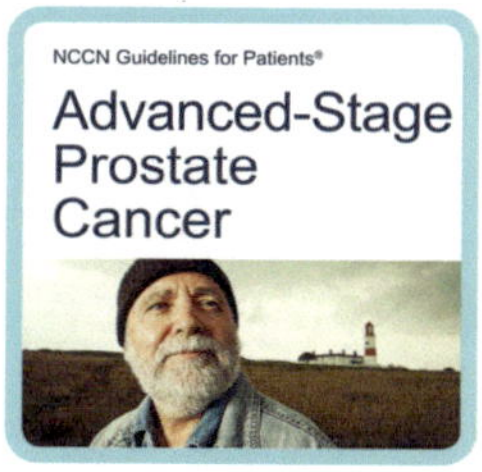

Biopsy result: No cancer is found

If your biopsy doesn't detect cancer cells in your prostate samples, it's called a negative result. But this is good news, because it means the biopsy **did not** detect cancer—it was "negative" for cancer.

Take time to enjoy the moment. Breathe a sigh of relief.

From now on, though, your doctor will want you to be on guard. You'll likely be advised to have regular prostate cancer screenings every 1 or 2 years. Your doctor may also recommend a biomarker test if you haven't had one already, and perhaps another mpMRI or even another biopsy depending on your risk.

Be sure to continue to go to follow-up visits, get tested regularly, and stay in touch with your doctors and health care team.

If your prostate cancer screening showed your PSA is higher than normal, you can have further testing and evaluation to get more information before undergoing a biopsy.

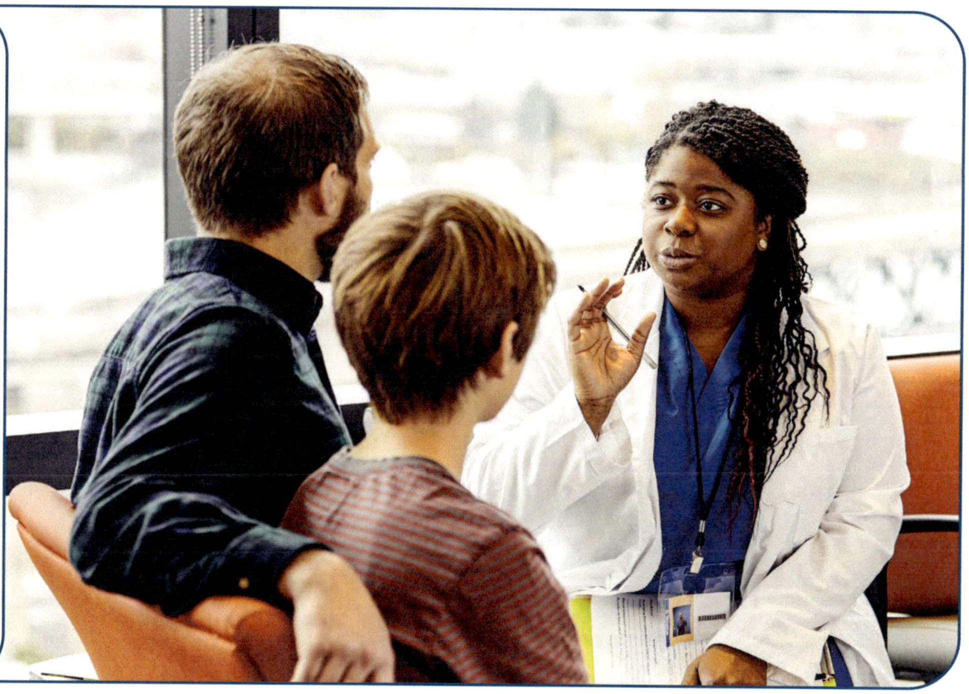

Key points

- Having a high level of prostate-specific antigen (PSA) doesn't mean you need to have a biopsy immediately. Experts recommend most people with a high PSA have other, noninvasive tests first.
- Most people who have a high PSA level should have another PSA test in a few weeks to verify the first test's results or to see if the PSA level has changed.
- Having an MRI before a biopsy can help you avoid getting a biopsy unnecessarily.
- An advanced type of MRI that's recommended for prostate cancer is called multiparametric MRI, or mpMRI.
- The only way to diagnose prostate cancer is with a biopsy.

Questions to ask

- How much of a change in my PSA level is considered significant?
- If I'm likely to need a biopsy, should I have an MRI first?
- How much time do I have to decide whether to have a biopsy?
- If I have 1 biopsy, will that be enough? Or does it mean I'll need to have more biopsies?
- If my biopsy finds prostate cancer, who can I talk to about next steps?

What's next?

If your biopsy finds cancer, don't panic just yet. Most cases of prostate cancer can be successfully monitored (watched without treatment) when found early, or treated if needed. If your biopsy doesn't detect cancer, take time to appreciate your life and enjoy your health. And remember to take care of your health by eating well, being active, and going to follow-up visits.

5 Other resources

Want to learn more? Here's how you can get additional help.

What else to know

This guide helps you know your options so you can make informed decisions and improve your cancer care. But it's not the only resource that you have.

Ask for as much information and help as you need. Many people are interested in learning more about:

- The specific details of prostate cancer screening and biopsies
- Talking with others who've gone through screening
- Prostate cancer diagnosis and treatment
- Health and nutrition recommendations to reduce prostate cancer risks

What else to do

Your health care center can help you with next steps. It often has on-site resources to help meet your needs and find answers to your questions. Health care centers can also inform you of resources in your community.

In addition to help from your providers, the resources listed in the next section provide support for many people like yourself.

Where to get help

Look through the list below and visit the provided websites to learn more about these organizations.

AnCan Foundation
ancan.org

CanCare, Inc.
cancare.org

Cancer*Care*
cancercare.org

Cancer Hope Network
cancerhopenetwork.org

Cancer Survivor Care
cancersurvivorcare.org

FORCE: Facing Our Risk of Cancer Empowered
facingourrisk.org

GRACE
cancergrace.org

Imerman Angels
imermanangels.org

Malecare
malecare.org

My Faulty Gene
myfaultygene.org

National Alliance of State Prostate Cancer Coalitions (NASPCC)
naspcc.org

Prostate Conditions Education Council (PCEC)
prostateconditions.org

Prostate Health Education Network (PHEN)
prostatehealthed.org

Triage Cancer
triagecancer.org

ZERO Prostate Cancer
zerocancer.org

We want your feedback!

Our goal is to provide helpful and easy-to-understand information on cancer. Take our survey to let us know what we got right and what we could do better.
NCCN.org/patients/feedback

Questions to ask

- Are you suggesting options other than what NCCN recommends? If yes, why?
- Can I get a second opinion on the results of my PSA test or MRI scan?
- Will I need PSA tests, digital rectal exams, and biopsies for the rest of my life?
- Is there financial assistance available for screening or biopsy?
- How can I connect with others who've been through prostate cancer screening?

Words to know

aggressive prostate cancer
Cancer of the prostate that grows or spreads quickly and often needs treatment right away. Also called high-risk or fast-growing prostate cancer.

biomarker
Something found in your body that can be measured to provide information about your health.

biopsy
A procedure that removes tissue samples to be tested for disease.

enlarged prostate
An overgrowth of tissue in the prostate that isn't caused by cancer. Also sometimes called benign prostatic hyperplasia.

erectile dysfunction
A lack of blood flow to the penis that limits getting or staying erect.

family history
Information about current and past health conditions that can reflect a pattern of certain diseases in a family.

life expectancy
The number of years a person is estimated to live based on statistics of other people in similar circumstances.

low-grade prostate cancer
Slow-growing, non-aggressive cancer contained within the prostate. It doesn't cause symptoms and rarely requires treatment. Also called low-risk prostate cancer.

magnetic resonance imaging (MRI)
An imaging test that uses radio waves and powerful magnets to make pictures of the inside of the body.

prostate exam
An exam of the prostate made by feeling it through the wall of the rectum. Also called a digital rectal exam.

prostate-specific antigen (PSA)
A protein made by the prostate that helps semen transport sperm.

PSA density
The level of PSA—a prostate-made protein—in relation to the size of the prostate.

PSA test
A blood test that measures the amount of PSA in your bloodstream.

risk factor
Something that increases the chance for getting a disease.

screening
A test (or tests) for finding signs of disease before having any symptoms.

shared decision-making
A process in which the doctor and the patient work together to make the best possible health care decision.

NCCN Contributors

This patient guide is based on the NCCN Clinical Practice Guidelines in Oncology (NCCN Guidelines®) for Prostate Cancer Early Detection, Version 2.2026. It was adapted, reviewed, and published with help from the following people:

Dorothy A. Shead, MS
Senior Director
Patient Information Operations

John Murphy
Senior Medical Writer

Lisa Diehl
Production Layout Artist

The NCCN Clinical Practice Guidelines in Oncology (NCCN Guidelines®) for Prostate Cancer Early Detection, Version 2.2026 were developed by the following NCCN Panel Members:

Preston C. Sprenkle, MD/Chair
Yale Cancer Center/Smilow Cancer Hospital

*Tyler M. Seibert, MD, PhD/Vice Chair
UC San Diego Moores Cancer Center

Kelvin A. Moses, MD, PhD/ Immediate Past Chair
Vanderbilt-Ingram Cancer Center

Clinton Bahler, MD, MS
Indiana University Melvin and Bren Simon Comprehensive Cancer Center

Geoffrey Box, MD
The Ohio State University Comprehensive Cancer Center - James Cancer Hospital and Solove Research Institute

William J. Catalona, MD
Robert H. Lurie Comprehensive Cancer Center of Northwestern University

Douglas M. Dahl, MD
Mass General Brigham Cancer Institute

Marc Dall'Era, MD
UC Davis Comprehensive Cancer Center

John W. Davis, MD
The University of Texas MD Anderson Cancer Center

Bettina F. Drake, PhD, MPH
Siteman Cancer Center at Barnes-Jewish Hospital and WashU Medicine

*Ruth B. Etzioni, PhD
Fred Hutchinson Cancer Center

Jonathan Fainberg, MD, MPH
Memorial Sloan Kettering

*Thomas A. Farrington, BSEE
Prostate Health Education Network, Inc.

Isla P. Garraway, MD, PhD
UCLA Jonsson Comprehensive Cancer Center

David Jarrard, MD
University of Wisconsin Carbone Cancer Center

Eric Kauffman, MD
Roswell Park Comprehensive Cancer Center

Deborah Kaye, MD, MS
Duke Cancer Institute

Adam S. Kibel, MD
Dana-Farber/Brigham and Women's Cancer Center

Chad A. LaGrange, MD
Fred & Pamela Buffett Cancer Center

Tamara Lotan, MD
Johns Hopkins Kimmel Cancer Center

Paul Maroni, MD
University of Colorado Cancer Center

*Brian Reys, MS, CGC
UT Southwestern Simmons Comprehensive Cancer Center

Simpa S. Salami, MD, MPH
University of Michigan Rogel Cancer Center

Alejandro Sanchez, MD
Huntsman Cancer Institute at the University of Utah

Terrence M. Shaneyfelt, MD, MPH
O'Neal Comprehensive Cancer Center at UAB

*Jonathan Shoag, MD
Case Comprehensive Cancer Center/ University Hospitals Seidman Cancer Center and Cleveland Clinic Taussig Cancer Institute

Abhinav Sidana, MD, MPH
The UChicago Medicine Comprehensive Cancer Center

Marc C. Smaldone, MD, MSHP
Fox Chase Cancer Center

Geoffrey Sonn, MD
Stanford Cancer Institute

Mark D. Tyson II, MD, MPH
Mayo Clinic Comprehensive Cancer Center

Neha Vapiwala, MD
Abramson Cancer Center at the University of Pennsylvania

Robert Wake, MD
St. Jude Children's Research Hospital/ The University of Tennessee Health Science Center

Samuel Washington III, MD, MAS
UCSF Helen Diller Family Comprehensive Cancer Center

Alice Yu, MD, MPH
Moffitt Cancer Center

Bertram Yuh, MD, MS
City of Hope National Medical Center

NCCN

Deborah Freedman-Cass, PhD
Senior Manager, Clinical Content Operations

Emily Kovach
Guidelines Layout Specialist

*Reviewed this patient guide. For disclosures, visit NCCN.org/disclosures.

NCCN Cancer Centers

For contact information, visit NCCN.org/cancercenters.

Abramson Cancer Center
at the University of Pennsylvania
Philadelphia, Pennsylvania

Case Comprehensive Cancer Center/
University Hospitals Seidman Cancer Center and
Cleveland Clinic Taussig Cancer Institute
Cleveland, Ohio

City of Hope National Medical Center
Duarte, California

Dana-Farber/Brigham and Women's Cancer Center |
Mass General Cancer Center
Boston, Massachusetts

Duke Cancer Institute
Durham, North Carolina

Fox Chase Cancer Center
Philadelphia, Pennsylvania

Fred & Pamela Buffett Cancer Center
Omaha, Nebraska

Fred Hutchinson Cancer Center
Seattle, Washington

Huntsman Cancer Institute at the University of Utah
Salt Lake City, Utah

Indiana University Melvin and Bren Simon
Comprehensive Cancer Center
Indianapolis, Indiana

Johns Hopkins Kimmel Cancer Center
Baltimore, Maryland

Mayo Clinic Comprehensive Cancer Center
Phoenix/Scottsdale, Arizona
Jacksonville, Florida
Rochester, Minnesota

Memorial Sloan Kettering Cancer Center
New York, New York

Moffitt Cancer Center
Tampa, Florida

O'Neal Comprehensive Cancer Center at UAB
Birmingham, Alabama

Robert H. Lurie Comprehensive Cancer Center
of Northwestern University
Chicago, Illinois

Roswell Park Comprehensive Cancer Center
Buffalo, New York

Siteman Cancer Center at Barnes-Jewish Hospital
and Washington University School of Medicine
St. Louis, Missouri

St. Jude Children's Research Hospital/
The University of Tennessee Health Science Center
Memphis, Tennessee

Stanford Cancer Institute
Stanford, California

The Ohio State University Comprehensive Cancer Center -
James Cancer Hospital and Solove Research Institute
Columbus, Ohio

The UChicago Medicine Comprehensive Cancer Center
Chicago, Illinois

The University of Texas MD Anderson Cancer Center
Houston, Texas

UC Davis Comprehensive Cancer Center
Sacramento, California

UC San Diego Moores Cancer Center
La Jolla, California

UCLA Jonsson Comprehensive Cancer Center
Los Angeles, California

UCSF Helen Diller Family Comprehensive Cancer Center
San Francisco, California

University of Colorado Cancer Center
Aurora, Colorado

University of Michigan Rogel Cancer Center
Ann Arbor, Michigan

University of Wisconsin Carbone Cancer Center
Madison, Wisconsin

UT Southwestern Simmons
Comprehensive Cancer Center
Dallas, Texas

Vanderbilt-Ingram Cancer Center
Nashville, Tennessee

Yale Cancer Center/Smilow Cancer Hospital
New Haven, Connecticut

Index

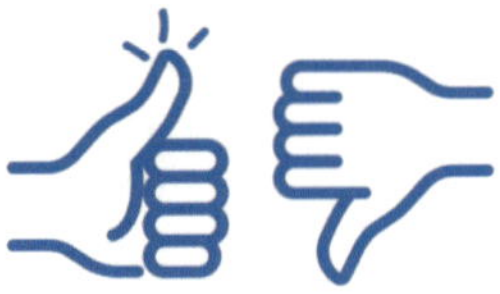

Let us know what you think!

Please take a moment to complete an online survey about the NCCN Guidelines for Patients.
NCCN.org/patients/response

Made in the USA
Monee, IL
05 November 2026

67382735R00024